medicine
and health

© Aladdin Books Ltd 1994

Designed and produced by
Aladdin Books Ltd
28 Percy Street
London W1P 9FF

First published in
the United States in 1994 by
Twenty-First Century Books
A Division of Henry Holt and Company, Inc.
115 West 18th Street
New York, NY 10011

Library of Congress Cataloging-in-Publication Data
Hawkes, Nigel
Medicine and health / Nigel Hawkes. – 1st ed.
    p. cm. – (New technology)
  Includes index.
  ISBN 0–8050–3417–X
  1. Medical innovations – Juvenile literature.
2. Medical technology – Juvenile literature.
I. Title. II. Series.
R855.4.H39 1994
610–dc20 94–6716 CIP AC

Design
David West
Children's Book Design
Designers
Edward Simkins
Flick Killerby
Editor
Jen Green
Research
Brooks Krikler Research
Illustrators
Alex Pang
Peter Harper

Printed in Belgium
All rights reserved

new TECHNOLOGY

medicine
and health

NIGEL HAWKES

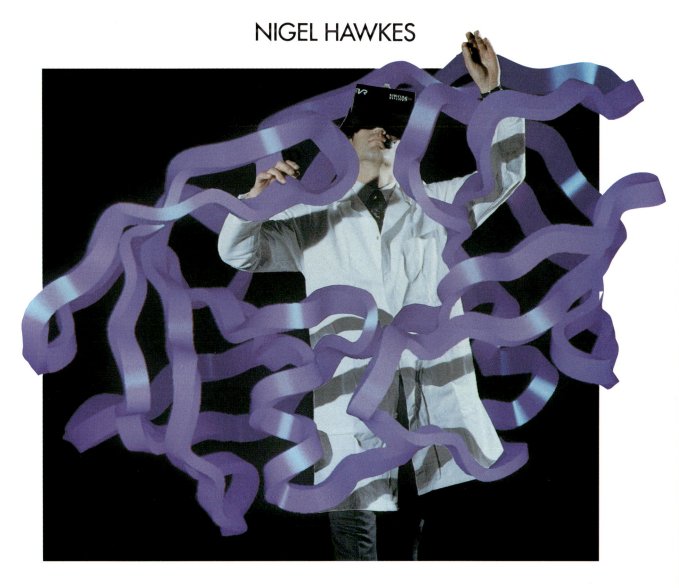

TWENTY-FIRST CENTURY BOOKS
A Division of Henry Holt and Company/New York

CONTENTS

INTRODUCTION	5
DIAGNOSIS	6
TESTING	8
GENE THERAPY	10
DRUG DESIGN	12
DRUG DELIVERY	14
SURGERY	16
LASER SURGERY	18
TRANSPLANTS	20
HEART REPAIR	22
IMPLANTS	24
FERTILIZATION	26
CHRONOLOGY	28
GLOSSARY	31
INDEX	32

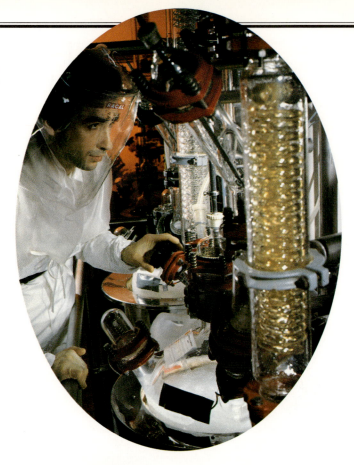

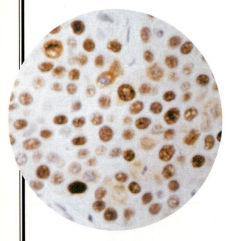

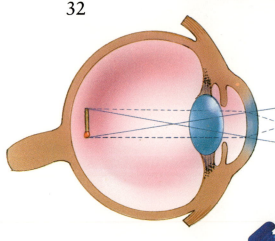

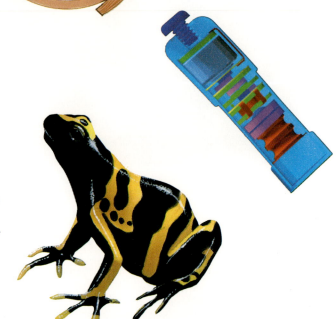

Photocredits
Abbreviations: t-top, m-middle, b-bottom, l-left, r-right
Front cover tl,14tr:Norplants Systems; cover tr & back: Medical Graphics & Imaging UCL; cover ml, 16t: Novosti Picture Library; cover bl, title p, 4t, 12t, 12-13: Glaxo Holdings PLC; 4m, 8b: Imperial Cancer Research; 4b, 10-11, 12b, 13-14, 14tl, 17mr & b, 24 both, 25tl & b: Frank Spooner Pictures; 6m, 7br, 10b, 11m & b, 13, 18-19, 19b, 21t, 23m, 25tr, 26t, 26-27, 27t, 29b, 30b: Science Photo Library; 6b, 6-7, 16-17: BUPA; 7t: Philips; 7bl: University College London; 8m, 8-9, 9t: Bayer; 14b, 27m: Roger Vlitos; 19t: Eastman Dental Hospital; 21bl & r: Imutran; 22-23: Thermo-Cardio Systems; 28 all, 29t & m, 30t & m: Hulton Deutsch.

INTRODUCTION
NEW TECHNOLOGY

The technology of medicine is advancing more rapidly than ever before. From heart transplants to artificial limbs, from gene therapy to laser surgery, doctors have new opportunities for prolonging life and curing disease. This book looks at the latest techniques in medicine, some so new they are still being tested. The battle against ill health will never end, because new diseases like AIDS emerge, and old ones learn new tricks to defeat the best drugs devised by medical researchers. But today's doctors possess resources that would have been undreamed of 50 years ago. Science has transformed the practice of medicine.

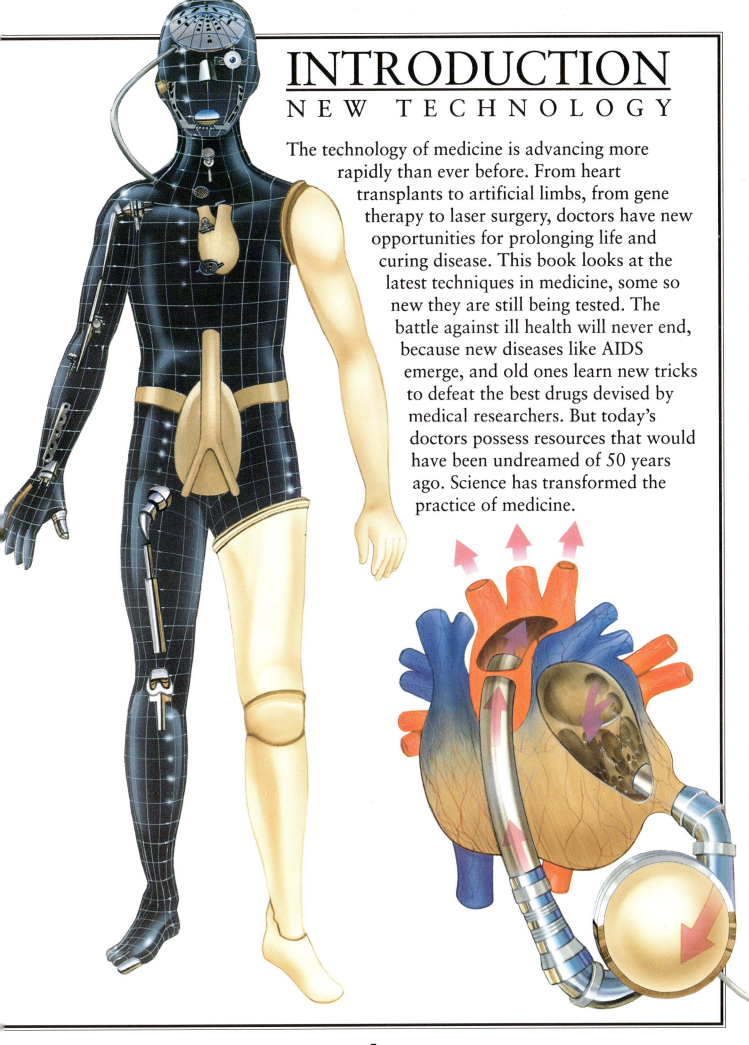

DIAGNOSIS
IDENTIFYING DISEASE

Before doctors can begin to cure they must correctly identify illnesses. Now new ways of seeing inside the body are improving diagnoses.

Better X-ray techniques and a new generation of scanners have transformed the pictures doctors have of their patients. Ultrasound, CAT, and MRI scans show the interior of the body in amazing detail, usually displayed on a computer screen. The MRI (magnetic resonance imaging) scanner, pictured right, monitors the behavior of atoms in the body when placed in a strong magnetic field. Doctors can also see directly into the body and carry out minor surgery using flexible telescopelike devices called endoscopes. The array of new diagnostic methods grows almost weekly.

MRI scanners (right) can see body parts in ever-improving detail. This image of a nerve in the wrist was produced by filtering out signals from fat and muscles that normally hide the nerves.

Ultrasound (left) produces images by detecting the echoes of high-frequency sound waves bounced from inner organs, like the sonar systems used for spotting submarines. It is ideal for checking babies growing in the womb.

A revolutionary laser scanning technique produced the 3-D computer image of a human face, shown opposite. Such images will help surgeons to perform the delicate work of facial reconstruction.

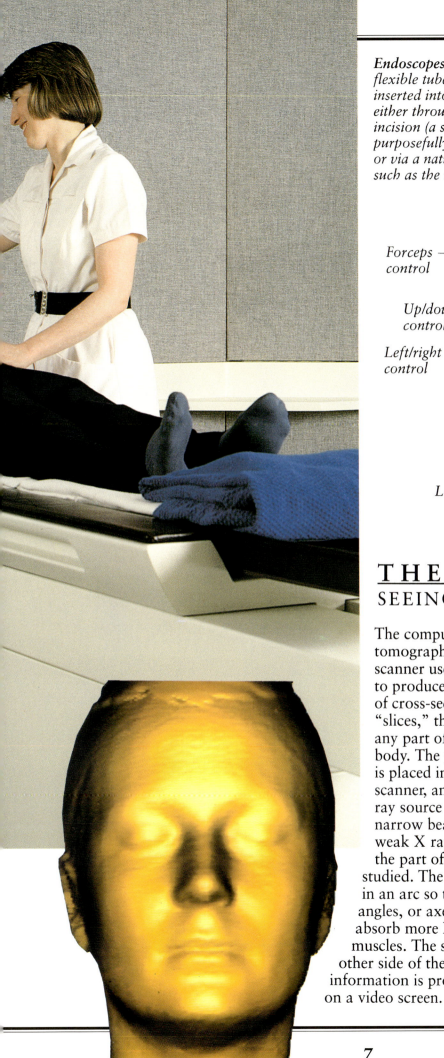

Endoscopes are long, flexible tubes that can be inserted into the body, either through an incision (a small purposefully made cut) or via a natural opening such as the mouth. Laser light passes along one fiber-optic channel in the tube, while another transmits the image. The surgeon can operate a miniature forceps, and blow in air to inflate an organ for a better view.

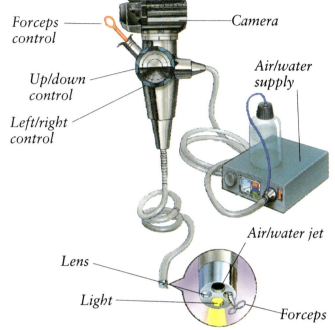

THE CAT SCANNER
SEEING THE BODY IN SLICES

The computerized axial tomography (CAT) scanner uses X rays to produce pictures of cross-sections, or "slices," through any part of the body. The patient is placed inside the scanner, and an X-ray source sends narrow beams of safe, weak X rays through the part of the body being studied. The source moves around in an arc so that the X rays come from various angles, or axes. Denser body tissues such as bone absorb more X rays than softer ones such as muscles. The strength of the rays emerging from the other side of the body is measured, and the information is processed in a computer and displayed on a video screen.

TESTING
BEFORE ILLNESS STRIKES

The chances of successful treatment are much greater if a disease is identified early – even before it produces symptoms. This has led to large-scale testing and screening for diseases such as breast and cervical cancer. In the future, we may do some of this screening ourselves, using diagnostic kits bought from the drugstore to check our blood pressure or blood sugar level. Sales of home diagnostic kits are booming, although some doctors are anxious about this development.

The handheld meter below shows the level of glucose in the blood, to help in controlling diabetes. A meter that would measure sugar levels in urine would be even simpler to use. Several companies are researching this idea.

The blood glucose test for diabetes shown right involves taking a tiny blood sample with a finger-pricking device, and then testing its glucose level. In diabetes, the body cannot use its blood sugars to provide energy, so there is a tendency for glucose to build up in the bloodstream.

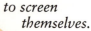

Some kits are designed not to detect a new disease but to follow the course of an established illness such as diabetes. People with certain types of diabetes must inject themselves regularly with insulin, which their bodies cannot make naturally, otherwise they may lapse into a coma. Home-testing kits can be used by people with diabetes to monitor their condition, and so improve control of the disease. This is important because if not properly treated, diabetes can lead to side effects such as blindness.

Cancer of the cervix (the neck of the womb) is a major killer, yet it can be detected early by the presence of abnormal cells in a sample called a cervical smear. Once found, there is a good chance of eliminating the cancer. Home tests might encourage more women to screen themselves.

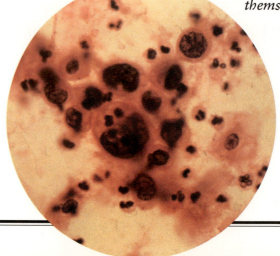

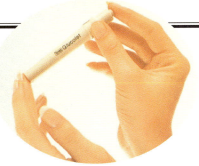

Cholesterol testing kits *(below) are among the most controversial available, because the results obtained vary. The kits monitor the level of the fatty substance* cholesterol in the blood. High levels are linked with an increased risk of heart attack, but smoking, obesity, and high blood pressure also increase the risk.

Pregnancy testing kits *and the blood glucose kits used by people with diabetes are the most successful home diagnostic kits. Diabetes is a very common condition, caused by the failure of the body to produce the hormone insulin, normally made by the pancreas.*

Home tests for AIDS have been produced, but are illegal in the United States. Doctors believe anyone being tested for the HIV virus that causes AIDS should receive counseling at the same time.

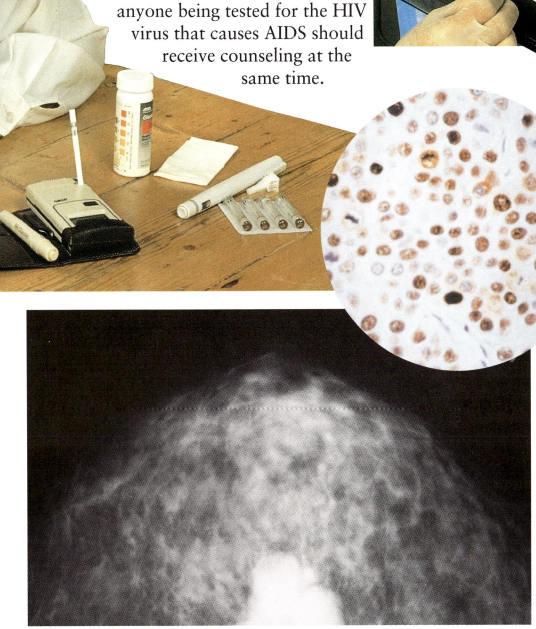

Breast cancer *is common in Western countries. Twelve percent of all American women will develop the disease, and 46,000 women die each year. Researchers have located a gene linked to breast cancer, P 53, here colored by a chemical stain in cancerous breast cells under the microscope.*

A lump in the breast *may be harmless – or it may be a cancerous tumor. Suspicious lumps can be detected by self-examination, then checked by an X ray, or by shining an infrared light through the breast. In Britain a national screening program has been introduced for women between 50 and 65, the age group most at risk.*

GENE THERAPY
BLUEPRINT OF LIFE

A new medical technique, gene therapy, is bringing hope to people suffering from genetic diseases.

Every cell in your body has its own "blueprint," a full set of instructions for building and maintaining the body. It is written as a chemical code in the molecules called deoxyribonucleic acid (DNA). A gene is a portion of DNA, that tells the cell what its job is. Mistakes in genes may arise haphazardly, as in Down's syndrome, or be inherited from parents, as in cystic fibrosis or muscular dystrophy. The idea behind gene therapy is to identify the faulty gene as early as possible and devise a way of replacing it with the correct version. One way is to attach the correct gene to a virus, and then allow the virus to "infect" the patient, getting right inside the body cells and carrying the correct gene with it. For safety reasons, the virus is made harmless so that it does not cause any illness during the "infection."

Each of the 60 trillion cells in your body contains a set of 46 chromosomes in its nucleus. Chromosomes consist of long, double spiral-shaped molecules called DNA.

The crosslinks between the spirals are made up of four different chemicals called nucleic acids, which contain the genetic code. On the right, a scientist examines fragments of DNA under ultraviolet light.

Humans have 46 chromosomes, two sets of 23 "twins," one set being inherited from each parent. Since each chromosome has a "twin," it is possible to have a defect in one chromosome without realizing it, because the other "twin" has the correct version. But when two people with the same defect have a child, the baby may inherit both defective copies, and manifest the genetic disease. Now that many of these genes are known, they can be detected before birth.

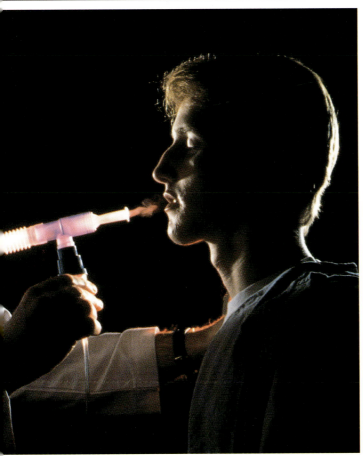

Cystic fibrosis is a genetic disease in which the gene for making fluid in the lungs is defective, causing frequent infections. Above, a researcher sprays a virus containing the correct gene into the lungs of a sufferer.

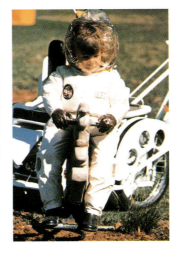

The first successful gene therapy patients were two girls in the United States. They had a rare genetic disease that makes the body vulnerable to infection. It is caused by lack of a gene that produces a body enzyme called adenosine deaminase (ADA). Such children survived in the past only if they were kept in a germ-free "bubble."

GENE SPLICING
HOW IT IS DONE

The photograph shown left shows how gene therapy helped the girls deficient in ADA. The technician controls a tiny needle, shown on the TV screen, which introduces the gene responsible for the production of the enzyme adenosine deaminase (ADA) into white blood cells. The cells were taken from the patients, and after the correct gene was inserted or "spliced" into them, they were returned, in the form of a bone marrow transplant. The white blood cells are the body's frontline against infection, attacking and killing germs. But they cannot function properly unless they can produce ADA. The girls are now living normal lives. Whether the treatment will need to be repeated regularly is not yet clear.

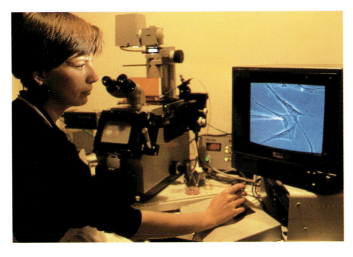

The right gene can be inserted into body cells by attaching it to a virus. Viruses pass into cells and take over their genetic machinery. Here a virus gene is snipped open, the new gene is spliced in, and then the virus is allowed to infect a cell.

DRUG DESIGN
TAILOR-MADE MEDICINES

Genetic engineering and new computer techniques are revolutionizing the manufacture of medical drugs used to treat disease.

Previously, many drugs were made by a process of trial and error. Research chemists produced new chemicals almost at random, and then tested them to see if they had any useful effects. In some cases, the researchers used natural products. But understanding how the body works now makes it possible to design tailor-made drugs. For example, knowing how the stomach makes acid for digesting food led to a new class of drugs that cut down acid production. This has helped millions of people who suffered from ulcers because their stomachs made too much acid. The gene revolution promises even greater successes. For example, suppose a disease is linked with a particular gene. From the structure of the gene and its genetic code, researchers can manufacture the substance that the gene should be producing, but isn't. So treatments can be devised to replace the missing substance.

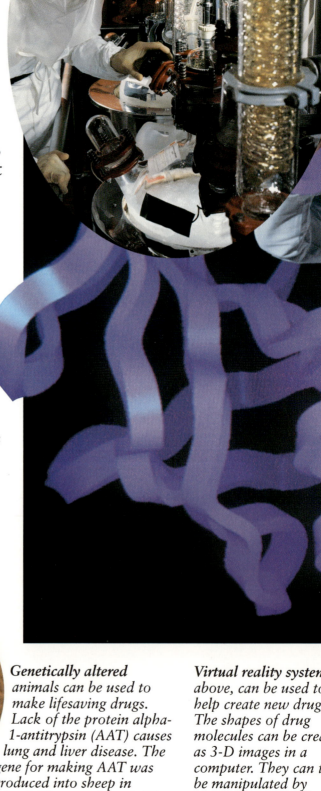

Genetically altered animals can be used to make lifesaving drugs. Lack of the protein alpha-1-antitrypsin (AAT) causes lung and liver disease. The gene for making AAT was introduced into sheep in Scotland. They produce AAT in their milk, for human patients.

Virtual reality systems, above, can be used to help create new drugs. The shapes of drug molecules can be created as 3-D images in a computer. They can then be manipulated by researchers to produce the most effective design.

The manufacture of drugs requires incredibly precise, controlled conditions. The photograph on the left shows a technician monitoring conditions during a critical stage in the manufacturing process.

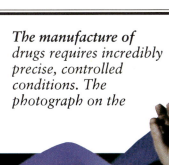

A frog from the Amazon region has long been used by native hunters. Its skin contains poisons for the darts used to immobilize the hunters' prey. Now the same chemical, in very small doses, may form the basis of a painkilling drug.

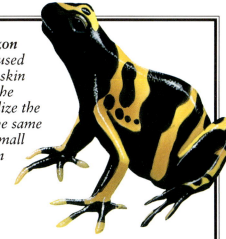

ANIMAL MEDICINES
REPRODUCING NATURE

Animals, plants, and fungi often provide the original versions of new drugs. Using genetic engineering methods, the relevant genes can be obtained from them and put into microbes, which then produce commercial quantities of the drug. A drug vital in the success of organ transplants, cyclosporine, was first found in fungi. It can now be manufactured synthetically. Snake venom has been tested to see if it can be "tamed" to produce useful medicines.

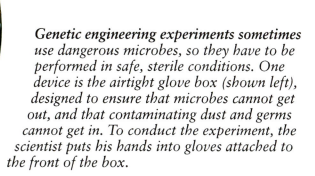

Genetic engineering experiments sometimes use dangerous microbes, so they have to be performed in safe, sterile conditions. One device is the airtight glove box (shown left), designed to ensure that microbes cannot get out, and that contaminating dust and germs cannot get in. To conduct the experiment, the scientist puts his hands into gloves attached to the front of the box.

13

DRUG DELIVERY
TARGETING DISEASE

New ways of getting drugs to the right place in the body could improve many treatments.

Cancer drugs are usually highly toxic, because they are designed to poison malignant cells. The trouble is that they also kill healthy cells. Targeting these drugs more accurately, so that they only reach the cancer and not the rest of the body, could improve their effectiveness. The easiest way to take a drug is by swallowing it, but this isn't always possible. Nanotechnology – the creation of microscopic machines – could provide a new approach. Minute capsules could find their own way about the body, until they reached the site of the disease, where they would release the drug. Another method would be to attach the drug to a natural body chemical such as an antibody, known to work at a specific site in the body.

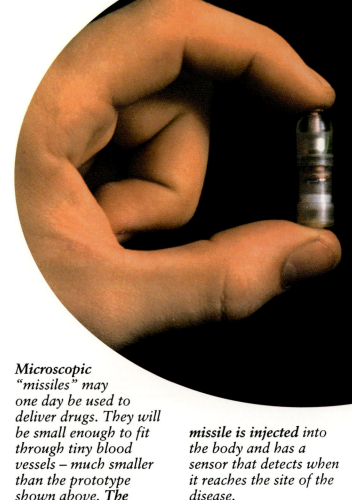

Microscopic "missiles" may one day be used to deliver drugs. They will be small enough to fit through tiny blood vessels – much smaller than the prototype shown above. The missile is injected into the body and has a sensor that detects when it reaches the site of the disease.

A new method of getting drugs to the right place is by attaching them to natural body molecules that guide them. One choice is an antibody molecule, one of the body's defenders against disease and germs. Antibodies attach themselves to the antigens on the surface of the germs. For cancer treatment, the poison ricin has been attached to an antibody known to seek out the cancer, and injected (1). When it gets to the cancer site (2), the poison is released to kill cancerous cells (3).

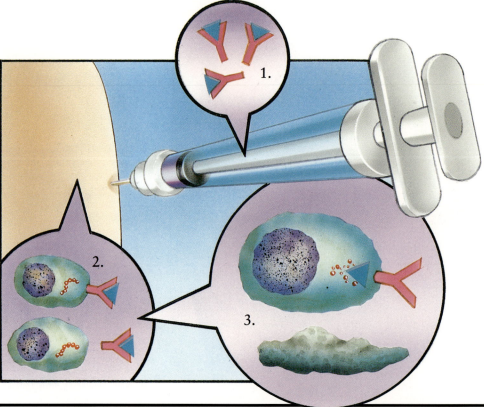

Contraceptive hormone chemicals are normally taken daily as pills. A new alternative is to make them in the form of strips that can be implanted just under the skin. The hormones in the strip seep into the body slowly. Such implants could be used for many other drugs.

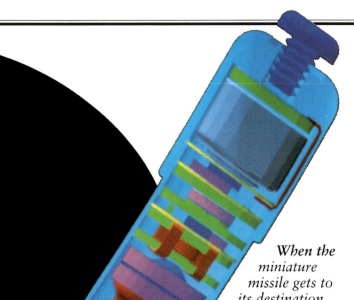

When the miniature missile gets to its destination, the sensor will trigger the release of exactly the right amount of the drug. Such missiles could also be used to measure chemicals and fluids in the body, and thus to diagnose disease.

Some drugs can be delivered from a skin patch, seeping through the skin and into the bloodstream beneath. Skin patches have helped some people to give up smoking. The patches contain nicotine, the addictive chemical contained in cigarette smoke. It finds its way through the skin, helping to satisfy the craving for a cigarette. The same technique has also been used to deliver drugs against seasickness and angina – a heart pain caused by narrowing of the coronary arteries in the heart. The patches can be stuck on the arms, chest, or just behind the ear.

A vaccination is the most effective way of prevnting many diseases. It prepares the body's immune system to fight a disease if it occurs. A vaccination may become available to fight one of the world's greatest killers, malaria. About three million people a year die of malaria, a tropical disease caused by a protozoan, which is passed on by mosquitoes. A Colombian scientist has developed a vaccine that mimics one stage of the disease. The vaccine contains a chemical copy of one of the body substances from the protozoan. In tests it has prevented infection in 40 to 60 percent of people. A major vaccination program could eliminate the disease.

15

SURGERY
SMALLER, QUICKER, NEATER

Once, major operations needed long incisions and left big scars. Today "keyhole surgery" has transformed many operations. Instead of cutting the patient wide open, the surgeon makes a small incision (the keyhole) and introduces an endoscope. This illuminates the interior of the body and transmits pictures that the surgeon can view on a screen. The operation is carried out through another small incision, using miniature surgical tools, or a laser (see pages 18-19). The major advantage is that small incisions heal quickly, so the patient makes a faster recovery. Keyhole surgery, correctly termed minimally invasive surgery, is now common for procedures such as repairing a hernia or removing the gallbladder. New surgical techniques do not have to go through exhaustive trials before they are introduced, so results have been variable.

Some illnesses previously requiring surgery can now be treated without an incision. Shock-wave lithotripsy is used for treating kidney stones. High-power shock waves of sound are beamed from outside the body at the stones. They shatter into tiny fragments, and pass out of the body through the urinary tract.

A keyhole operation for removing gallstones in the gallbladder, next to the liver, is shown right. The surgeon operates a mini-laser that destroys the stones. The surgeon is monitoring progress on a video screen that shows the inside of the patient, illuminated by the endoscope. Keyhole surgery makes totally new demands on surgeons, since the operation can be viewed only via the screen.

In some keyhole operations, a small slip would lead to serious problems, perhaps causing internal bleeding. Learning to "look away" and watch the screen while making delicate movements is a difficult skill to master. Devices that can make the task easier are needed.

The Robodoc system could enable the skills of an experienced surgeon to be transmitted across the world. The surgeon has handset controls that are connected to a computer. The computer transmits the surgeon's commands via satellite to the operating room, where robot arms wielding surgical instruments precisely carry out the commands. The surgeon monitors progress on a video screen, and assistants in the operating room check the patient and change the robot's instrument attachments.

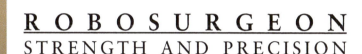

ROBOSURGEON
STRENGTH AND PRECISION

The Robodoc system pioneered by Dr. William Bargar and Dr. Howard Paul of Sacramento, California (below) could transform operations such as hip replacements, which require great strength as well as skill. The hip replacement operation (see page 24) involves the insertion of

Rather than looking up at a video screen, surgeons using a system designed in Ohio have the image in front of their eyes. They wear a helmet like a bicycle safety helmet, with a small color video screen mounted on it. All members of the surgical team can wear a helmet, giving them all a perfect view.

a metal pin with a rounded head, which fits inside a plastic socket bonded to the patient's hip bone. The pin is traditionally driven in by force, sometimes causing the bone to splinter. Robodoc's computer can produce 3-D images of the hip area and drill the cavity for the pin with great accuracy. In the future the system could also be used in precision ear, eye, and brain surgery.

17

LASER SURGERY
MAKING LIGHT WORK

The intensely bright, powerful, pure light of laser beams is finding more and more applications in medicine. Lasers can cut or burn off unwanted tissue neatly and quickly. They seal small blood vessels as they go, so bleeding is much reduced. Their greatest success has been in a new operation, to reshape the cornea at the front of the eye. This corrects near or far sightedness. Lasers are also used for other eye operations, and for destroying cancerous tumors, stopping ulcers from bleeding, and for removing birthmarks or tattoos. Different types of lasers produce different light, suitable for specific jobs. Carbon dioxide lasers are used for precise cutting and neodymium lasers for destroying tumors close to nerves. Lasers are even replacing drills in some dental surgeries.

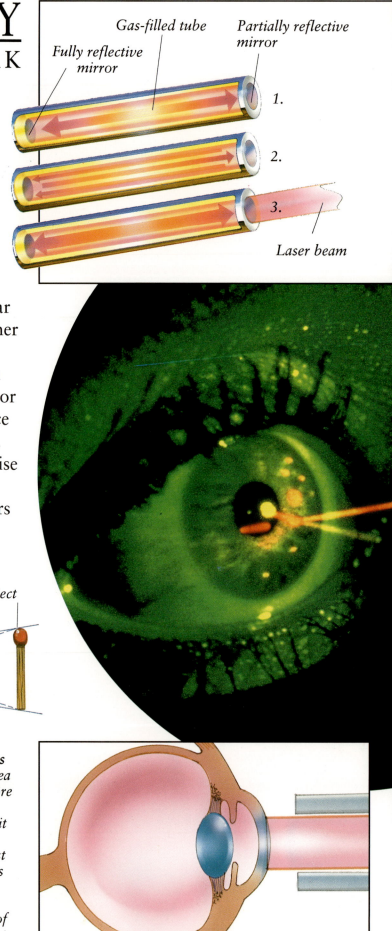

Near sightedness (above) occurs when the eyeball is too long for the focusing power of the cornea and lens. Light falling on the eye is focused not on the light-sensitive retina, but in front of it. The eye sees a blurred scene.

Laser surgery weakens the power of the cornea to focus light. The more curved a lens is, the more focusing power it has. To reduce the cornea's power, it must be made flatter. This is done by burning a precisely calculated amount off the front of the cornea with a burst of laser light.

The laser uses the properties of atoms or molecules to produce a powerful beam of pure light. The laser tube (shown opposite) contains a mixture of gases. An electrical charge can be used to give energy to atoms in the gas. This "excites" the atoms, causing them to fire off photons – tiny bursts of light. The photons collide with other atoms, making them fire off photons too. The photons bounce back and forth along the laser tube between the mirrors at both ends (1). With each pass, the intensity of the light increases (2), until finally it is powerful enough to burst through the partial mirror at the front of the laser, to form the laser beam (3).

By far the greatest medical use of lasers is in eye surgery. The first operations to correct near sightedness were pioneered in Russia. One method, radial keratotomy, involved making a series of fine scalpel cuts in the cornea, radiating outward like the spokes of a wheel. As the cuts healed, the cornea shrank slightly and became flatter, thus improving vision. The method worked, but was difficult to control. It has largely been replaced by the laser, which can remove precisely calculated slices from the cornea in a safe and predictable way.

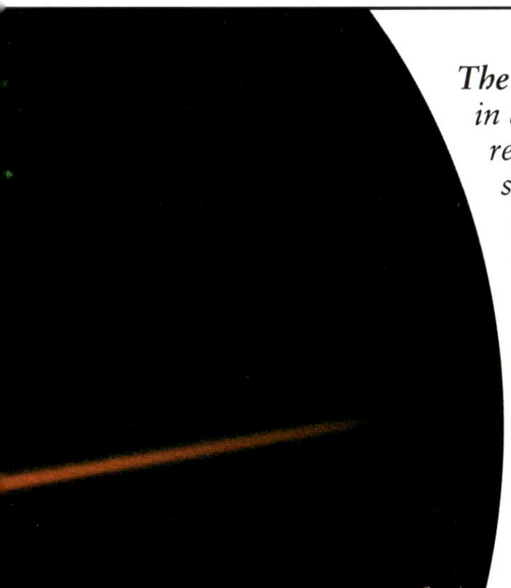

The laser is also used in dentistry. It can replace the high-speed rotary drill for cleaning holes and cavities in teeth before filling (shown right), and apparently produces no pain. Laser dentistry is becoming common in the United States.

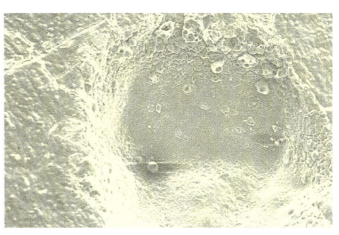

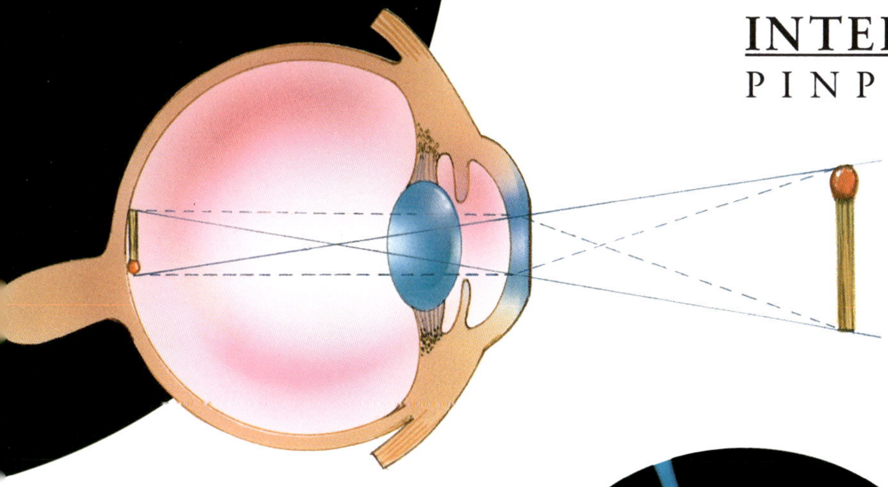

INTERNAL OPERATIONS
PINPOINT ACCURACY

The intense beam of a laser can be used to make an incision with absolute accuracy. For internal operations, lasers are combined with endoscopes (see page 7). Laser beams travel along the endoscope and can be shone exactly where the surgeon wishes. Lasers have been used to destroy gallstones (see page 16), and to cut away fatty deposits in the heart's coronary arteries that may lead to heart attacks. Argon lasers could be used in brain surgery (demonstrated left), to locate a tumor and vaporize it, while minimizing damage to surrounding tissue. One advantage of the laser is that there is no danger of infection from contaminated needles.

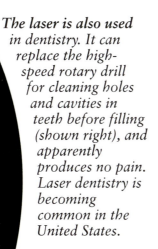

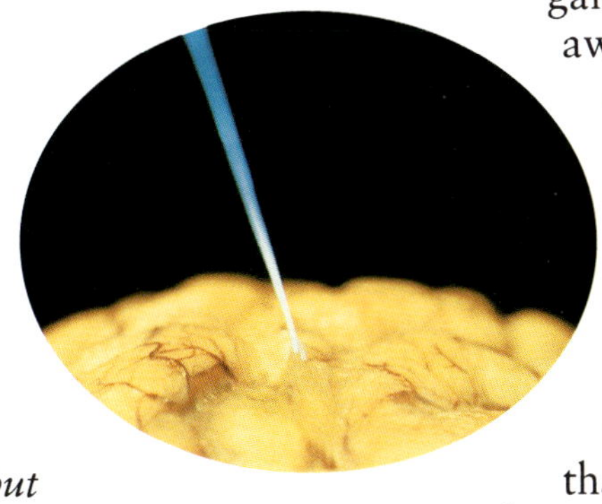

After surgery (above) the light comes to a precise focus at the retina. Many people treated no longer need their glasses, though this cannot be guaranteed. Lasers can also be used to treat far sightedness. The cornea is reshaped to make it more curved and thus increase its focusing power. This operation is an exciting development but not yet well-proven.

TRANSPLANTS
NEW PARTS FOR OLD

An organ is a major part of the body, such as the heart or liver. Transplanting organs from donors to recipients has been one of the success stories of modern medicine. When the first heart transplant was carried out in 1967, the patient died after 18 days. Today at least two-thirds of heart transplant patients survive for five years. Methods are improving all the time. In California, a young patient whose lungs had been destroyed by cystic fibrosis was saved when her parents each donated a single lobe from the five in their own lungs, to be transplanted into her chest.

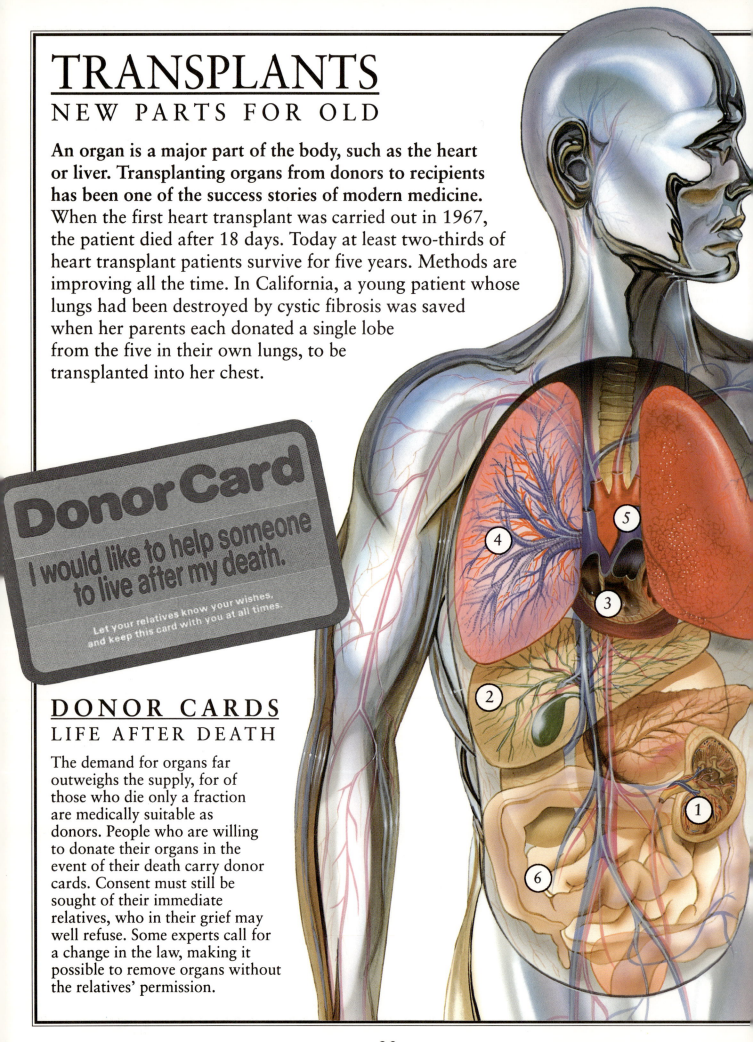

DONOR CARDS
LIFE AFTER DEATH

The demand for organs far outweighs the supply, for of those who die only a fraction are medically suitable as donors. People who are willing to donate their organs in the event of their death carry donor cards. Consent must still be sought of their immediate relatives, who in their grief may well refuse. Some experts call for a change in the law, making it possible to remove organs without the relatives' permission.

One of the obstacles to successful transplant surgery is rejection – the process by which the body recognizes and destroys "foreign" tissue. Better drugs to control rejection are now being made. Another major limitation to some transplants is that someone must die to provide an organ before someone else can be saved. The exception is kidneys, the organs that filter and clean the blood. The body has two kidneys, so one can be transplanted from a living donor. Kidneys are among the easiest organs to transplant. They are relatively simple to remove and replace, and can be preserved for 24 hours in a life-support machine like the one shown right.

1. Kidneys: a total of 1,766 kidney transplants were carried out in Britain in 1992; there were 4,464 patients on the waiting list.
2. Liver: the second most commonly transplanted organ, with 506 in 1992 and 83 on the waiting list.
3. Heart: 340 transplants, 325 on the waiting list.
4. Lungs: 89 transplants, 145 on the waiting list.
5. Heart/lung: 53 transplants, 236 waiting.
6. Intestine: rare.

Kidneys are the most commonly transplanted organs, but they also have the longest waiting list. This is because a person with kidney disease can be kept alive on a kidney dialysis machine while waiting for an organ. If a person's liver fails, they cannot be kept alive, so the waiting list is short. In some heart transplants the lungs are transferred as well, since there are fewer vessels and tubes to join. Among future possibilities are nerve transplants, designed to restore nerves damaged in accidents.

One answer to the shortage of organs could be animals. Normally, when an animal's organs are transplanted into a human, they are rejected in a matter of minutes. Now scientists in the United States and Britain, including John Wallwork and David White from Cambridge, below, are genetically engineering animals so that their organs have human proteins on their surface. These proteins should "turn off" the recipient's rejection system, enabling the transplanted organs to survive. The first trials are expected within five years.

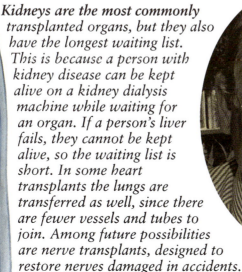
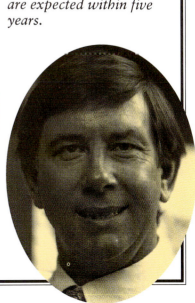

HEART REPAIR

HELPING BLOOD PUMP

Heart disease kills more people in the developed world than any other condition. But new drugs and surgical techniques have begun to cut the toll. The main cause of heart disease is the buildup of fatty lumps, called atheroma, in the coronary arteries that supply the heart's muscle with blood. Surgeons can replace blocked arteries with veins taken from the leg, or clear out the arteries to allow the blood to flow freely again. Pacemakers can steady an erratic heartbeat, and artificial valves replace damaged heart valves.

The ThermoCardio System is a pump that can be connected to the left side of the heart. Made of titanium, the inside of the pump has a rough surface. This encourages living blood cells to settle on it, forming a layer that helps the blood to flow freely. Power for the artificial heart is electrical, transmitted by coils mounted inside and outside the body.

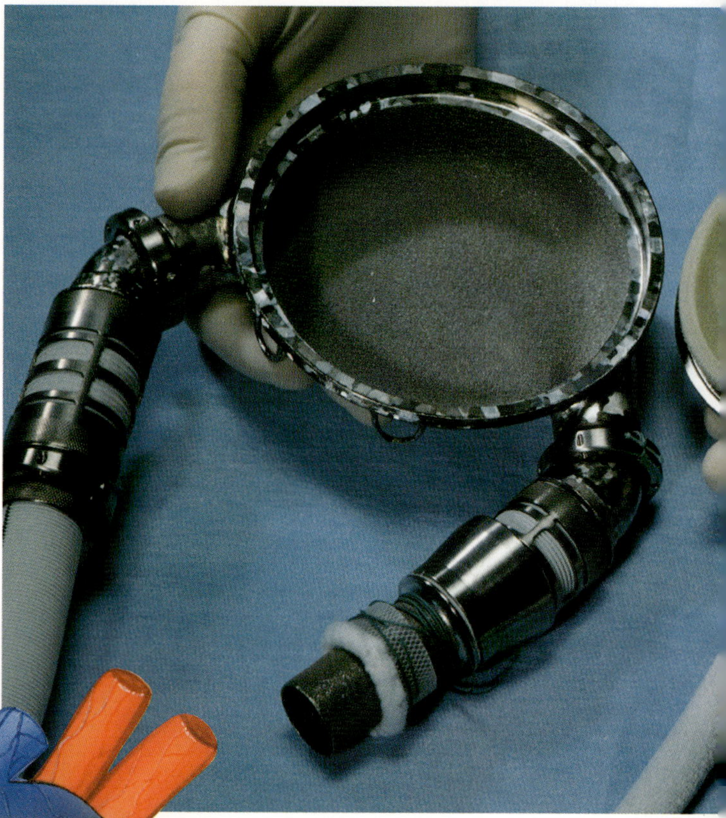

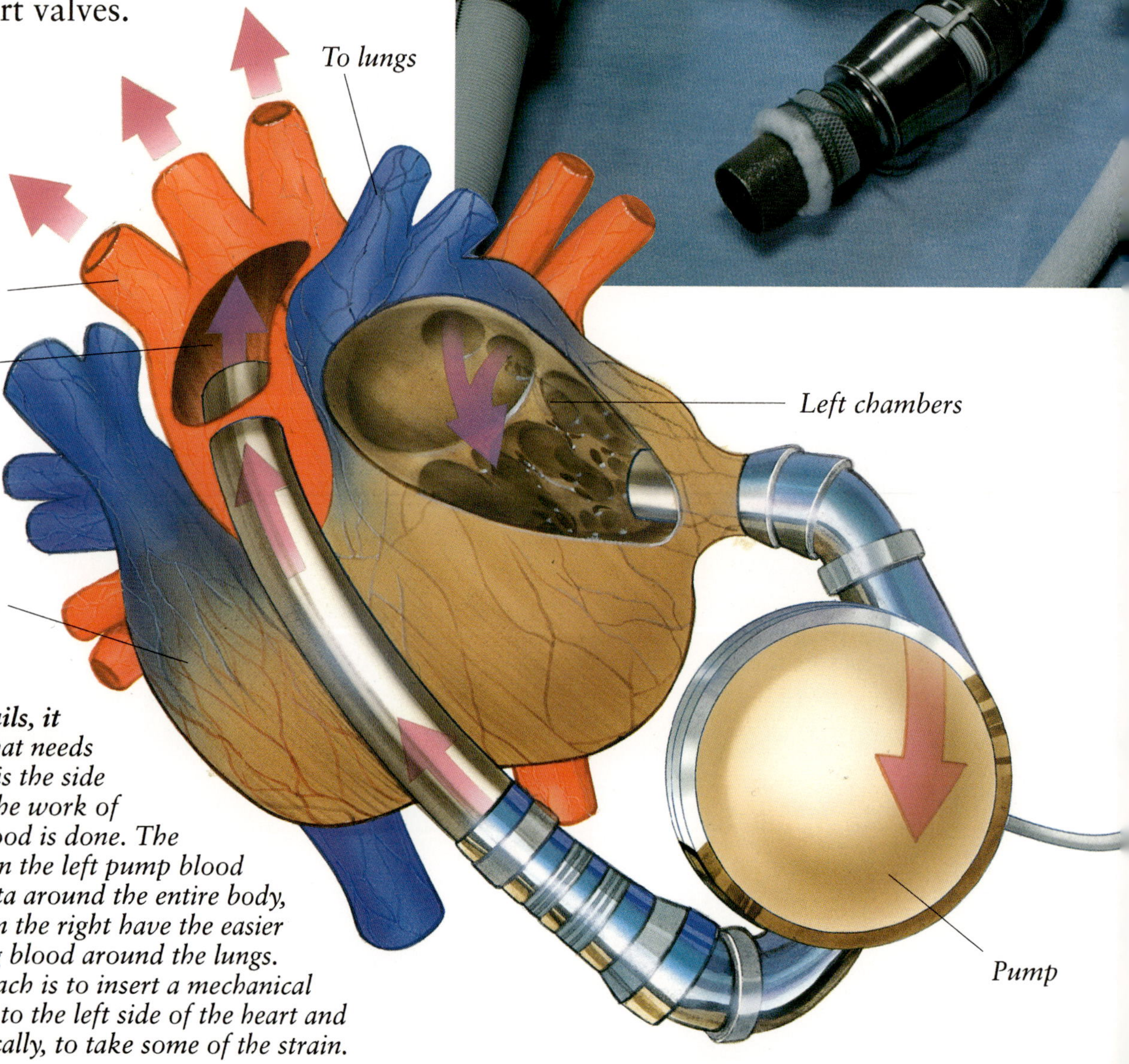
To lungs
To body
Aorta
Left chambers
Right chambers
Pump

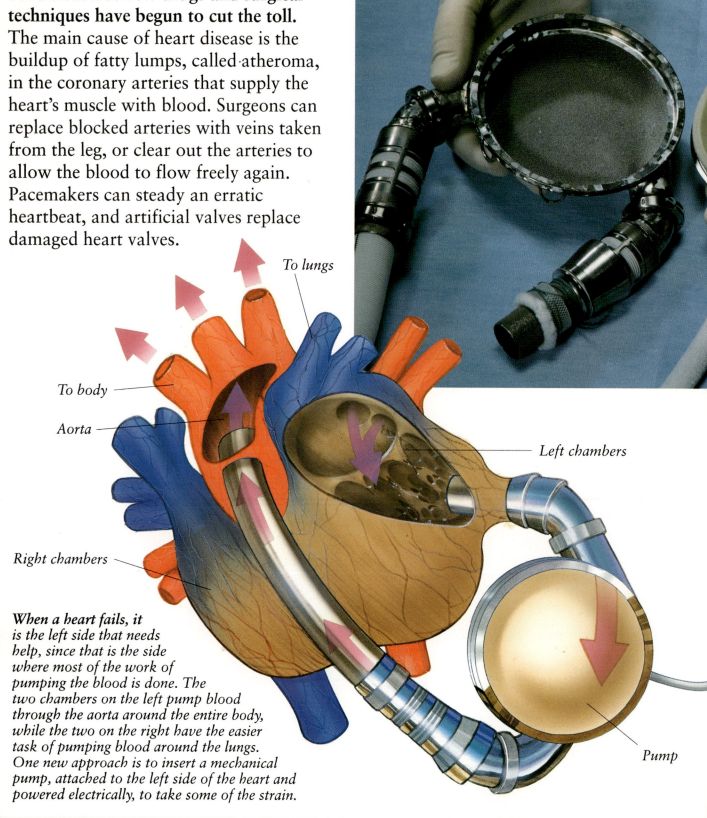

When a heart fails, it is the left side that needs help, since that is the side where most of the work of pumping the blood is done. The two chambers on the left pump blood through the aorta around the entire body, while the two on the right have the easier task of pumping blood around the lungs. One new approach is to insert a mechanical pump, attached to the left side of the heart and powered electrically, to take some of the strain.

A new technique for restoring blood flow to damaged heart muscle uses a laser to punch tiny holes in it. The holes stop bleeding quickly, but not before oxygen-rich blood has found new ways to flow through the muscle, thereby creating new blood vessels. 12 to 15 holes are made.

Laser

Heart muscle

Smoking and diets high in animal fats seem to contribute to the buildup of fatty deposits in the coronary arteries. Once the blood flow is restricted, the heart has to work harder to pump blood around the body, causing a pain called angina. The heart muscles may be starved of oxygen-bearing blood, permanently damaging them. Drugs called beta-blockers steady the heartbeat, ease pain and reduce the risk of heart attack. Blood-thinning drugs called "clot-busters," and humble aspirin, are also effective in treating heart problems.

MUSCLE GRAFT
AIDING THE HEART

Unlike the liver, which can gradually recover from injury and certain illnesses, damaged heart muscle cannot repair itself and regenerate. The normal treatments aim to make the job of pumping easier, by thinning the blood, widening the arteries, and changing the patient's diet. But the new technique of grafting shoulder muscle may be able to restore the heart's pumping power. The shoulder soon recovers its former strength.

A coronary bypass operation grafts new arteries onto the heart to replace those that have become narrowed or blocked. During the operation the machine in the foreground above is used to pump the patient's blood while the heart undergoes surgery.

The big muscle in the *shoulder, the latissimus dorsi (1), can repair the heart. Part of the muscle is removed, with its blood supply (2), and rolled into a tube (3). This fits around the blood vessel leading to the heart (4). It is connected to a pacemaker, (5) which triggers it into regular contractions, in time with the heart itself.*

IMPLANTS
SPARE-PART SURGERY

Surgeons estimate that within 50 years one person in ten will have at least one artificial part inside them.

The materials first used to make artificial parts included wood and gold. Today's bioengineers have a vast range of metals, plastics and other "inert" substances that the body will not reject. Some of the most commonly implanted artificial parts are hip, knee, ankle, and shoulder joints, which banish the pain and stiffness caused by arthritis. Steel plates and pins are used to hold broken bones in place and aid rapid healing. Artificial blood vessels of woven plastic fibers replace arteries damaged by disease, and robotic hands now provide increasing dexterity.

The silicon chip would be inserted in the eye behind the lens, so that light was focused onto it. Signals from the chip would pass along the optic nerve to the brain.

SILICON CHIP
RESTORING SIGHT

The retina of the human eye detects light rays shining on it and responds by sending electrical nerve signals to the brain. In certain forms of blindness the retina does not respond in this way. In the future a silicon chip could replace the retina and enable some blind people to see. The thumbnail-sized chip would be connected directly to the optic nerve that leads to the brain. Similar artificial eyes could be used for surveillance, to recognize faces, as shown on the left.

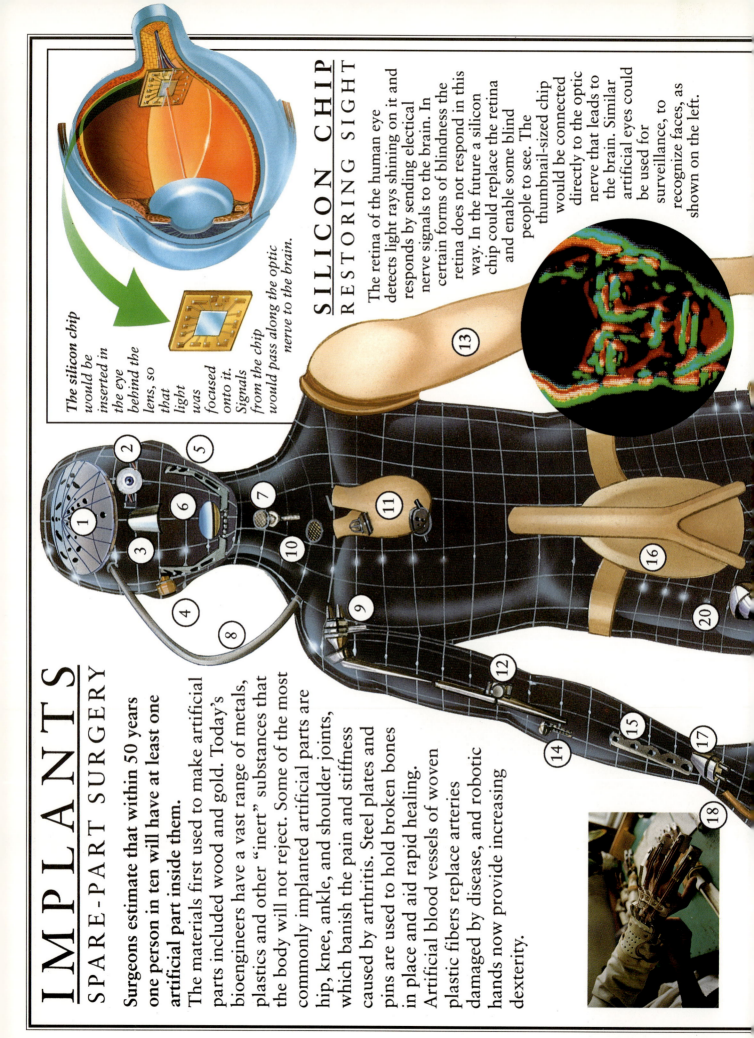

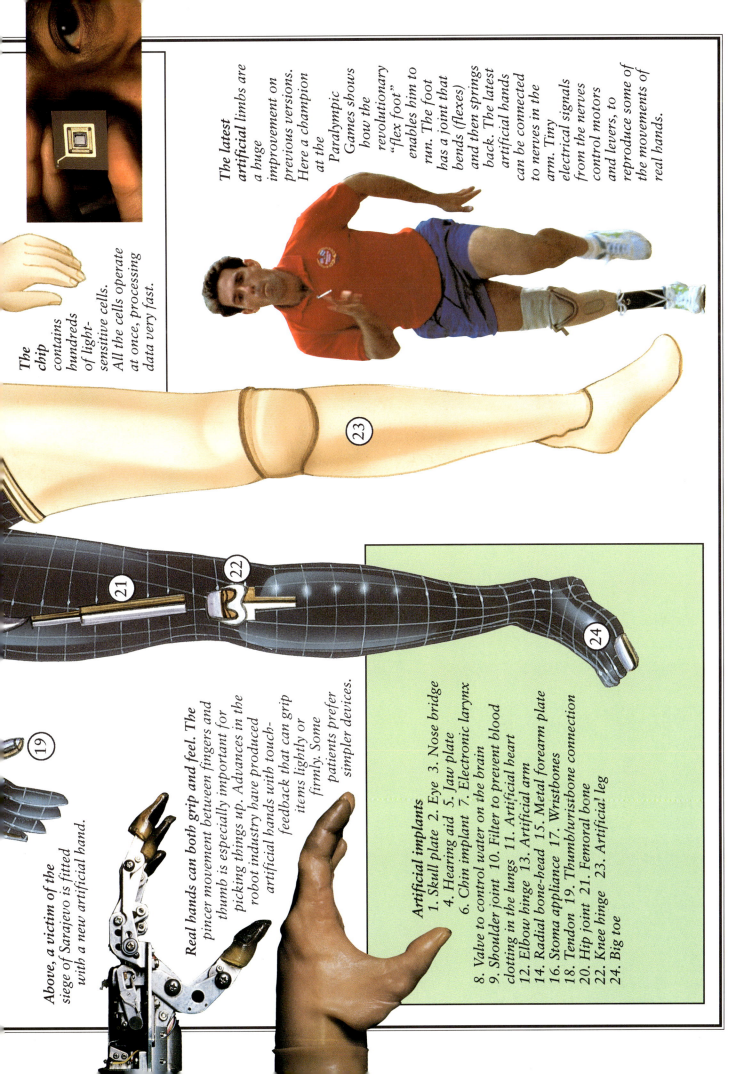

The latest artificial limbs are a huge improvement on previous versions. Here a champion at the Paralympic Games shows how the revolutionary "flex foot" enables him to run. The foot has a joint that bends (flexes) and then springs back. The latest artificial hands can be connected to nerves in the arm. Tiny electrical signals from the nerves control motors and levers, to reproduce some of the movements of real hands.

The chip contains hundreds of light-sensitive cells. All the cells operate at once, processing data very fast.

Real hands can both grip and feel. The pincer movement between fingers and thumb is especially important for picking things up. Advances in the robot industry have produced artificial hands with touch-feedback that can grip items lightly or firmly. Some patients prefer simpler devices.

Above, a victim of the siege of Sarajevo is fitted with a new artificial hand.

Artificial implants
1. Skull plate 2. Eye 3. Nose bridge
4. Hearing aid 5. Jaw plate
6. Chin implant 7. Electronic larynx
8. Valve to control water on the brain
9. Shoulder joint 10. Filter to prevent blood clotting in the lungs 11. Artificial heart
12. Elbow hinge 13. Artificial arm
14. Radial bone-head 15. Metal forearm plate
16. Stoma appliance 17. Wristbones
18. Tendon 19. Thumb/wristbone connection
20. Hip joint 21. Femoral bone
22. Knee hinge 23. Artificial leg
24. Big toe

FERTILIZATION
MAKING BABIES

About one couple in ten who want to have a baby is infertile. Techniques now exist to help many of these couples. In vitro fertilization (IVF) – literally, fertilization in glass – was first used successfully in Britain in 1978 to help women with one of the most common infertility problems: blocked fallopian tubes. These are the tubes along which the ripe egg cells normally travel from the ovary where they are made, to meet the sperm cells from the man, for fertilization. In IVF, ripe eggs are removed from the woman's ovary by an endoscope technique called laparoscopy. They are placed in a shallow glass dish (despite the popular name "test-tube baby," test-tubes have never been used). In the dish sperm from the man are added to fertilize the eggs, which are then returned to the woman's womb to develop in the normal way. An alternative method is not to let the sperm fertilize the eggs out of the body, but to return them all to the lower part of the fallopian tube, beyond the blockage.

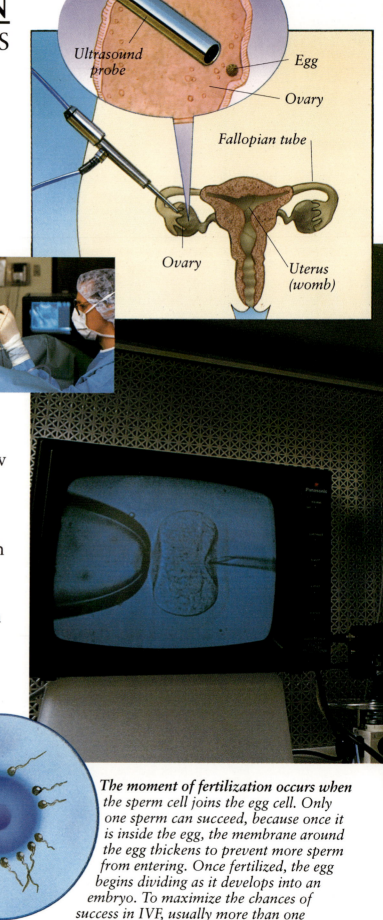

The ripe egg is surrounded by an outer membrane called the zona pellucida. Normally sperm can penetrate this layer to fertilize the egg. In some cases the sperm may not be strong enough, or the layer may be unusually thick. If so, a microinjection technique can be used. A very fine-pointed needle is used to penetrate the zona pellucida and inject the sperm. Developed in Italy, this method has achieved many successes.

The moment of fertilization occurs when the sperm cell joins the egg cell. Only one sperm can succeed, because once it is inside the egg, the membrane around the egg thickens to prevent more sperm from entering. Once fertilized, the egg begins dividing as it develops into an embryo. To maximize the chances of success in IVF, usually more than one fertilized egg is placed in the womb.

Ripe eggs are removed from the ovaries by inserting a laparoscope (see photo and diagrams opposite). The woman will have taken a fertility drug to ensure that she produces enough ripe eggs. Signals from a fine ultrasound probe produce images of the ovary and eggs. The eggs are sucked up through a very fine tube inside the laparoscope.

In some cases, the man produces too few sperm, or sperm that are too weak, to fertilize the egg. IVF may incorporate a technique for directly injecting the sperm into the egg. Once the fertilized eggs begin to develop into very early embryos, they can be frozen and stored for later use. In 1987-1988, test-tube twins were born in Britain 18 months apart, from embryos created on the same day.

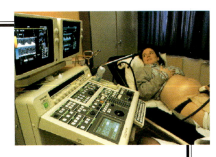

Before the baby is born, the developing embryo and mother are carefully scanned using ultrasound (see page 6) to check that all is well. The scan allows doctors to check the baby's progress.

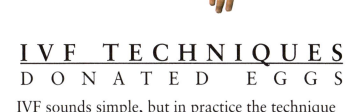

IVF TECHNIQUES
DONATED EGGS

IVF sounds simple, but in practice the technique has many difficulties. In the first ten years of the treatment in Britain, only one woman in ten who underwent IVF actually gave birth to a healthy baby. More controversial still is a technique for producing pregnancies in much older women, who are well past natural child-bearing age. This uses IVF with eggs donated by a younger woman. In Italy, women as old as 63 have had babies following this technique. But it is discouraged or even illegal in other countries, where IVF clinics will not carry it out.

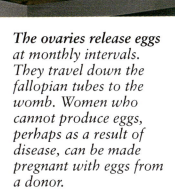

The ovaries release eggs at monthly intervals. They travel down the fallopian tubes to the womb. Women who cannot produce eggs, perhaps as a result of disease, can be made pregnant with eggs from a donor.

CHRONOLOGY

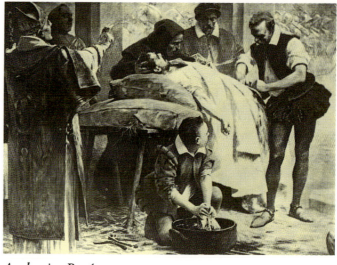

400 BC Hippocrates, the greatest of the Greek doctors, produced the basis of modern medical ethics, the Hippocratic Oath.
300 BC Chinese practiced acupuncture, and had a pharmacy of more than 2,000 different treatments, mostly herbal.
129 Galen, a Greek physician who practiced in Rome, began the study of anatomy, and made the first attempts to apply scientific observation to medicine.
1100 The first medical schools opened in Europe.
1286 The first post-mortem examination was carried out, in Cremona.
1543 The first accurate anatomical textbook was published by Andreas Vesalius.
1563 Ambroise Paré, a French surgeon, pioneered many important advances, including the use of artificial limbs and the tying off of arteries to prevent bleeding.
1628 The English doctor William Harvey described the circulation of the blood and the heart's role as a pump.
1657 The first practical syringe was invented in England.
1665 The first blood transfusion from one animal to another was performed by the English doctor Richard Lower.
1676 Using a microscope, the Dutch scientist Anton van Leeuwenhoek discovered that a drop of water teems with living creatures.
1733 Stephen Hales measured blood pressure in animals and humans.
1735 The first successful removal of the appendix was performed by the English military surgeon Claudius Amyan.
1753 James Lind, a doctor from Scotland, showed that the symptoms of scurvy could be alleviated by fresh fruit.
1796 Edward Jenner proved that smallpox could be prevented by vaccinating people with cowpox. The discovery was the beginning of the science of immunology.
1800 Chlorine was used for the first time to purify water.
1816 René Laënnec invented the stethoscope for listening to sounds from within the chest.
1826 The endoscope, which enabled the interior of the body to be examined, was invented by the French doctor Pierre Segalas.
1844 Horace Wells, an American dentist, first used nitrous oxide as an anesthetic.
1846 William Morton, also an American dentist, pioneered the use of ether as an anesthetic.

Ambroise Paré

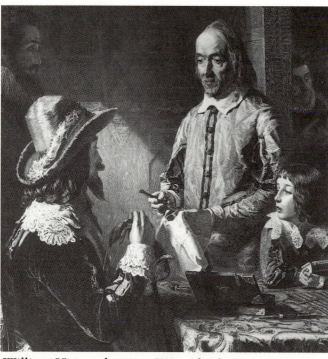

William Harvey lectures King Charles I.

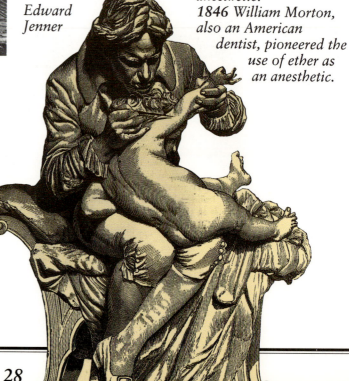

Edward Jenner

1847 Chloroform was first used as an anesthetic, in Britain.

1847 The Hungarian Ignaz Semmelweis showed that puerperal fever, a common disease in childbirth, could be eliminated by thorough disinfection.

1854 John Snow proved that cholera is carried by polluted drinking water.

1859 Charles Darwin's Origin of Species proposed a theory of evolution by natural selection.

1862 Louis Pasteur proposed that diseases are spread by germs, microscopic organisms passed by contact or through the air.

1865 The English surgeon Joseph Lister introduced antiseptic surgery, using carbolic acid to kill germs.

1866 The Austrian monk Gregor Mendel founded the science of genetics with his experiments on sweet peas.

1876 Robert Koch, a German doctor, proved that the disease anthrax is caused by rod-shaped bacteria called bacillae. He showed too that these bacteria could be grown in a culture outside the body.

1881 Pasteur successfully vaccinated animals against anthrax.

1890 Surgeons at Johns Hopkins Hospital in Baltimore began using rubber gloves for operations, a practice that soon became widespread.

1895 Within weeks of the discovery of X rays by Wilhelm Roentgen, doctors were using them to examine bone fractures.

1899 The drug aspirin was first marketed by the German chemical company Bayer. Today 100 billion aspirin are taken every year.

1905 Ernest Starling described the actions of hormones.

1905 The Austrian ophthalmologist Eduard Zirm carried out the first cornea transplant.

1909 Paul Ehrlich and Sukehachiro Hata, after testing 606 different compounds, discovered Salvarsan, a cure for the sexually transmitted disease syphilis.

1921 Insulin was isolated and used to treat people with diabetes.

1928 Alexander Fleming discovered penicillin from a mold in a culture dish left on the windowsill of his laboratory in London.

1941 Penicillin was finally used in medicine, after Howard Florey and Ernst Chain, at Oxford, found how to isolate it from the mold discovered by Fleming.

1943 American microbiologist Selman Waksman discovered streptomycin, a cure for tuberculosis.

1951 The contraceptive pill was developed by Gregory Pincus in the United States.

1953 The first open-heart surgery was performed at Jefferson Medical College at Philadelphia by John Gibbon, using a machine to take over the functions of heart and lungs.

1953 Francis Crick and James Watson worked out the structure of the genetic material DNA.

1954 The first successful kidney transplant was performed, in Boston.

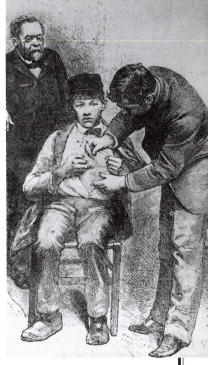

Louis Pasteur

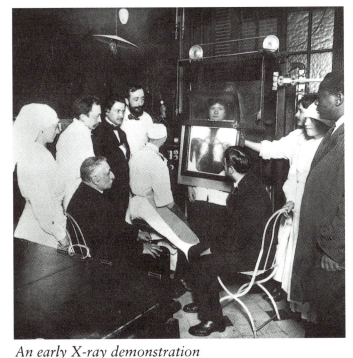

An early X-ray demonstration

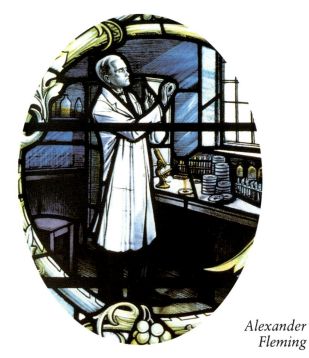

Alexander Fleming

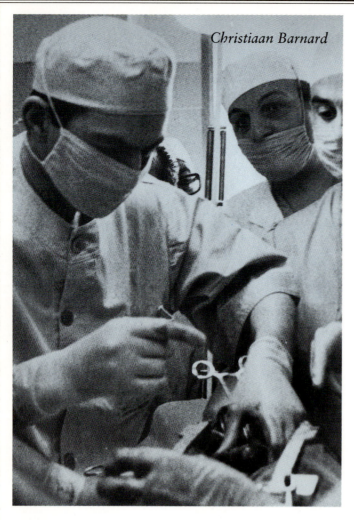
Christiaan Barnard

1955 Jonas Salk developed a polio vaccine.
1958 Ultrasound was developed to examine unborn children, by Ian Donald, a Glasgow doctor.
1958 The cardiac pacemaker was invented by the Swedish doctor Ake Senning.
1964 Charles Daughter, an American doctor, conducted the first angioplasty operation, inserting a tiny balloon inside an artery and blowing it up at the point where the artery was narrowest.
1967 The first heart transplant was performed in South Africa by surgeon Christiaan Barnard.
1967 Coronary bypass surgery, using veins taken from other parts of the body to replace coronary arteries damaged by disease, was attempted by surgeon René Favaloro in Cleveland.
1969 The first permanent artificial heart, inserted into a human patient in the U.S., kept him alive for three days.
1972 Computerized brain-scanners were developed by Godfrey Hounsfield of Britain.
1973 Magnetic resonance imaging was developed at Aberdeen University.
1973 Recombinant DNA technique for introducing foreign DNA into bacteria was discovered.
1975 Monoclonal antibodies were developed by César Milstein, in Britain.
1975 Smallpox was eliminated by mass vaccination campaigns organized by the World Health Organization: a great success in preventive medicine.
1978 The first baby fertilized in a "test tube" was born.
1982 Three German doctors developed a way of breaking down kidney stones by the use of shock waves.
1984 Luc Montagnier at the Pasteur Institute in Paris and Robert Gallo of the U.S. National Institutes of Health all found the cause of AIDS – acquired immuno-deficiency syndrome. It was the HIV virus.
1985 Minimally invasive, or "keyhole" surgery was developed.
1990 The gene for cystic fibrosis, the most common single gene defect, was isolated.
1993 Trials of gene therapy to try to cure the defective gene in patients suffering from cystic fibrosis began.
1994 First trials of AIDS vaccines began.

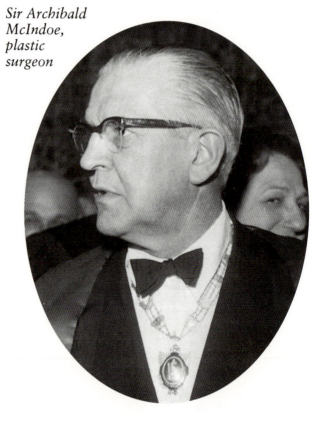
Sir Archibald McIndoe, plastic surgeon

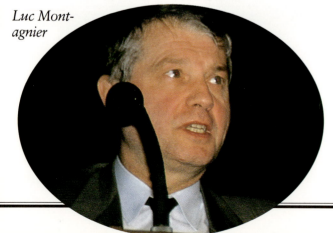
Luc Montagnier

GLOSSARY

Antibody
A protein produced by the body's white blood cells that recognizes a foreign substance, such as a bacterium.

Antigen
The foreign substance that stimulates production of antibodies. It could be a germ or a transplanted organ.

Arthritis
Inflammation of the joints, causing pain and restricting movement.

Cholesterol
A compound made by the liver and found in many tissues in the body. High levels of cholesterol in the blood seem to increase the risk of heart attack.

DNA
A molecule that contains all the genetic information passed on from parents to offspring.

Endoscope
A long fiber-optic tube through which light can pass, used for seeing inside the body. The stomach, for example, can be viewed by passing an endoscope down the throat.

Gallstones
Solid objects formed in the gallbladder by the formation of crystals. They can cause infections and block the bile duct.

Hormones
Chemical messengers made by the glands that circulate through the body, regulating natural body processes such as digestion, growth, and sexual development.

Lithotripsy
The technique of breaking up kidney and gallstones by beaming powerful shock waves at them from outside the body.

Nerve
Cord-like fibers specialized to carry messages, in the form of tiny electrical signals. Nerves coordinate most body processes.

Neuron
A cell found in the brain, specialized to conduct nerve impulses.

Organ
A part of the body with a distinct function, such as the heart or the liver.

Penicillin
The first antibiotic drug able to kill bacteria in the body.

Vaccine
A material injected or swallowed into the body that mimics the process of infection, thus instructing the body to produce antibodies. When the real infection comes along, the body is prepared and is able to resist it.

INDEX

AIDS 9
acupuncture 28
adenosine diaminase (ADA) 11
anesthetic 28-29
anthrax 29
antibody 14
antigen 14
antiseptic surgery 29
appendix 28
arthritis 24

blood transfusion 28
brain surgery 19

cancer 14, 18
  breast 8, 9
  cervical 8
cervical smear 8
cholera 29
cholesterol testing kit 9
chromosomes 10-11
contraceptive pill 29
cyclosporine 13
cystic fibrosis 10, 11

dentistry 18, 19
DNA (deoxyribonucleic acid) 10
diabetes 8, 29
diagnosis 6-7
donor card 20
Down's syndrome 10
drugs 12-15, 21, 29
  design 12-13
  targeting disease 14-15

endoscope 6, 7, 16, 19, 28

eyes
  silicon chip 24
  surgery 18, 19

gallstones 19
gene therapy 10-11
genetic engineering 12-13, 21

heart
  angina 15
  attack 9, 19, 23
  muscle graft 23
  open-heart surgery 29
  pacemaker 22, 30
  ThermoCardio System 22
hernia 16
hip replacement 17, 24
history of medicine 28-30
home-testing kits 8-9
hormones 15, 29

identifying disease 6
implants 17, 22, 24-5, 28, 29
in vitro fertilization (IVF) 26-27

keyhole surgery 16
kidney stones 16

laser surgery 16, 23
  argon 19
  carbon dioxide 18
  neodymium 18

malaria 15

muscular dystrophy 10

nanotechnology 14-15
nerves 6, 21

open-heart surgery 29
organs 13, 20-21, 29, 30

penicillin 29
polio 30
pregnancy testing kits 9

Robosurgeon 17

scanners 6, 30
  CAT (computerized axial tomography) 6
  MRI (magnetic resonance imaging) 6, 30
  ultrasound 6, 27, 30
screening 8-9
shock-wave lithotripsy 16
smallpox 28, 30
streptomycin 29
syphilis 29

transplant surgery 13, 20-21
  cornea 29
  heart 20, 21, 30
  kidneys 21, 29
  liver 21
  lungs 20, 21
tuberculosis 29
tumors 18, 19

vaccination 15, 28, 30
virus 11, 20